Weight Loss Success

Books about Weight Management

Susan Kersley

Published by Susan Kersley, 2021.

WEIGHT LOSS SUCCESS

First edition. April 18, 2021.

Copyright © 2021 Susan Kersley.

ISBN: 979-8201201272

Written by Susan Kersley.

Table of Contents

Are you ready to shed your excess weight? 1

Overweight is not good for you....................................3

Do you really want to lose weight? 5

Why bother? 6

What to avoid when you want to lose weight....................................8

What to do when you want to lose weight.................... 11

Five keys to success 13

Eat breakfast to lose weight 15

Carbohydrates, do you need them?.................... 16

Don't want to follow a strict eating programme?.................... 18

Exercise for weight loss 19

The best diet is one that you devise for yourself.................... 22

Weight loss – the importance of where you are.................... 24

Eat less and exercise more.................... 26

What is the best way to do this? 27

Eat regularly 29

What is vital for your good health and well-being?.................... 30

Think about your daily routine.................... 32

Get a more positive approach to weight loss.................... 33

Eating behaviour 34

Diets don't work... 35

Ways to lose weight without dieting................................ 37

Weight loss and good intentions 39

How to regain the weight you lost 40

How to get your weight loss back on track..................... 42

How to maintain your weight loss 45

Exercise.. 47

More about exercise.. 49

Unhealthy versus healthy 51

Finally.. 53

Are you ready to shed your excess weight?

———

You know you would feel and look much better if you lost some weight. Not only that but your health and well-being would improve too. However, for one reason or another you haven't been able to get into the right mindset to achieve what you want.

What can you do to make this the time you really do become the weight you'd like to be and shed the excess fat for ever?

1. Be absolutely clear about the changes you want to make and what will be involved. Take it step by step. Set small goals and achieve them. For example, you might decide not to have so much bread or stop eating sweet biscuits. Or you might add more fruit and vegetables to your meals and avoid putting such a big portion on your plate.

2. What will you start doing? You could change your mindset about food and become more aware of exactly what you are putting into your mouth. The best foods to eat are those cooked or uncooked which are as near to their natural state as possible.

3. What will you stop doing? You might stop buying a bar of chocolate to eat on the way home from the supermarket. Or stock up your cupboard with low fat protein foods such as chicken and fish. You could stop using so much oil in food preparation.

4. Who else will be affected by your changes?

The person you live with might not want to stop eating certain foods.

What will happen if you take no action and you carry on as before? Your weight will continue to increase and eventually your health may suffer the effects of obesity.

5. Are you ready to take the next step?

Have you decided what your long-term goal around your health and well-being is? It doesn't have to be about the weight you want to be. It could be instead about how you feel, what you can do which you can't do now and what sort of energy you will experience.

If you want to change your weight, you have to develop a clear vision of how life would be for you as a slimmer person so that what you come to terms with the way you will be able to do things you find challenging now. You will be able to wear different styles of clothes too and have more energy to enjoy life much more.

Are you prepared to make plans, develop workable strategies for change and then take actions required?

Overweight is not good for you

You've finally decided that it's time to do something about your weight. However, you know that diets don't work because you've tried so many. You lose some weight only to put back the same and more when the diet is 'over' and you start eating 'normal' food.

Losing weight, in the long term, is more about your mindset than trying to stick to a diet formula. You can't live the rest of your life counting calories or adding up points. It's not realistic.

What you must do instead is to make your everyday diet as healthy as possible and change your habits around eating.

The first thing to do is to look through your food cupboard and freezer and get rid of all the food that you know is not good for you, because if you no longer have unhealthy foodstuff readily available you won't eat it.

Then you need to change your food buying habits. This process is easier if all members of your household help you towards achieving the goal of healthy eating since it will not only be you who will benefit from more healthy food. They will be healthier if they, and you, eat less sugar and more fruit, vegetables, lean protein and fish.

Changing your eating and food-buying habits will result in you eating more wholesome food and this is an important step in your progress towards attaining a more healthy weight.

It may be the time of the year or it may be big family celebration that means you've eaten more lavishly than usual and not stuck quite so rigidly to your healthy eating. Now you want to lose weight in a healthy and long term beneficial way.

Many of the population of Great Britain and the United States of America are grossly overweight. The blame for this may be due to doing less exercise and eating high sugar and highly processed foods that become addictive: the more of them you eat the more you want.

Take yourself in hand and resolve to eat less or cut out completely highly processed food and decide it's the right time to exercise on a regular basis and eat more unprocessed food.

Do you really want to lose weight?

If you eat too much, eat unhealthy food and fail to exercise then you will continue staying overweight. If you want another outcome then you have to do something differently.

The result of not changing anything will be in twenty, thirty- or forty-years. When you are eighty years old will you then turn around and say, 'OK now I'm ready. Now I have the time to eat more healthily, do more exercise and find other ways to respond to emotions instead of overeating'.

Do you know how to change?

When you are sure you really want to be slimmer, you already know the formula: *'Eat less, eat more healthily and exercise more.'*

Are you going to apply the changes?

You know the outcome you want and what to do. Now you must take action.

To help you decide whether now is the right time for change, ask yourself these important questions:

- What will happen if I do?

- What will happen if I don't?

- What won't happen if I do?

- What won't happen if I don't?

Why bother?

There is a lot of talk about how many of the population in the Great Britain, and in the United States of America are grossly overweight. This is true and a lot of the blame for this may be in relation to a lot of us doing less exercise and eating high sugar and high fat foods that almost become addictive: the more of them we eat the more we want to eat them.

We need to take ourselves in hand and resolve to eat less if not cut out completely these sorts of food and decide its the right time to exercise on a regular basis and eat more food in as much as possible in it's unadulterated state.

Why should you be bothered to keep your weight within a healthy range? Here are five reasons why you should do that.

To reduce the risk of heart disease

It is well known that being overweight increases your risk of high blood pressure, stroke and heart attacks. Of course, some people, unlucky enough to suffer any of these conditions, are not overweight, but you reduce your chances by being a healthier weight.

To reduce the risk of diabetes

Similarly type 2 diabetes is more likely to develop in those who are overweight. Diabetes can lead to developing other serious medical complications.

To be able to move easily

It's more difficult to be agile when you are overweight. Movement and exercise are important to keep your body in the best shape. Overweight and exercise are interconnected: when you weigh too much it's more difficult to exercise, yet when you exercise you will lose the excess weight more easily.

To have a greater choice in what to wear

More choice of clothes is a good reason to lose excess weight.

To live longer

If you are within a healthy weight range you are less likely to develop life limiting conditions. Not being ill means a greater chance for a longer and healthier life. No one can predict how long you will live but however long that is, it's better to be healthy and in good shape for as long as possible.

What to avoid when you want to lose weight

L osing weight isn't easy and there are thousands of books telling you what to do, but it can be a challenge.

So how can you make it easier on yourself to avoid temptation to eat more than you want and need to eat?

1. Takeaways

When you're tired and don't feel like preparing your own meals it's very tempting to buy a takeaway. Of course, once in a while is fine because balance in all things is a good principle to live by. However, they are likely to be very high fat and extremely high calorie, neither of which do you want if you are attempting to lose weight.

Avoid the need for takeaways by making sure you have ingredients at home with which you can prepare a quick nutritional and not fattening meal very quickly. For example, if you have a microwave, some potatoes and a time of baked beans or a carton of cottage cheese you can make a meal in less than ten minutes.

2. Getting too hungry

It's better for your general health and your weight-loss journey especially, if you avoid going for long periods of time without any food. If you have a small snack in between meals, you will maintain your blood sugar at a good level and be able better to resist eating too much when you get to the next meal. Suitable healthy snack might be a piece of fruit with a few nuts or an oatcake or rice cake with a thin spread of peanut butter.

3. Too much alcohol

Alcohol is best kept to a minimum when you are trying to lose weight because not only does it have a calorie value without any nutritional benefit but if you have excessive alcohol you make either be depriving yourself of essential nutrients or be less likely to make suitable decisions about what to eat or what to avoid.

4. Ready prepared meals

You needn't avoid these completely and having a few of these in your freezer might be a good alternative to having a takeaway. However, avoid having them regularly because they tend to be have high fat and high salt. So read the labels carefully so you are more aware of their nutritional value, if any.

5. Easy access to unhealthy and fattening foods.

If you don't buy it then you are less likely to eat it! If you want to cut down your intake of biscuits, cakes and sweets then don't buy any.

What to do when you want to lose weight

You know you are overweight and plan to go on another diet or eating plan to try to lose some of your excess weight once and for all. But what to do? There are so many confusing plans all persuading you that theirs is the only way to finally become slim and healthy.

However, there is no secret formula. There is a simple way to become healthier and lose your excess fat, though you might find this difficult to accept. What you have to do is eat less and exercise more. It's a simple matter of arithmetic. If you are bigger than you want to be then this balance isn't correct. Which applies to you?

Even if you believe that your diet is healthy then there will be another factor coming into play.

It may be because although you eat healthy food, you eat too much of it. To achieve this you could reduce the size of your portions so that your intake is less or decide not to have a second helping. It is said you eat with your eyes, so you can fool yourself into believing you are eating more than you think by using a smaller plate and or piling high the low-calorie high bulk foods such as vegetables and salad.

Eat more fruit and vegetables and less high calorie foods.

For example, eating avocado pear is a very healthy choice. it has good fat and plenty of vitamin E. But it has a lot of calories. So, you have to strike a balance weighting up how healthy a food is against how many calories it has.

To contrast you might know that a spoonful of sweet jam has less calories than half an avocado. Nutritionally it contains a large quantity of sugar so is not so beneficial for your health as an avocado even though it has less calories.

Similarly with nuts such as walnuts or almond which are good for your health, contain healthy fat but are high in calories. So have some, perhaps a handful each day for your health but no more to reduce your calorie intake.

Another way to lose weight is simply to write down everything you eat during the day. This enables you to discover ways to eat less but strangely enough even the act of recording what you eat seems to mean that you change your eating habits and as a result lose your excess weight.

Five keys to success

It may be the time of the year or it may be big family celebrations which mean you've eaten more lavishly than usual and not stuck quite so rigidly to your healthy eating rules. Now you want to lose weight in a healthy and long-term beneficial way.

Here are five keys to being successful.

Get into the mindset for weight loss

Relax several times every day for a minute or two and let the tension go from your body as you breathe in relaxation. Tell yourself you are breathing in willingness and motivation to succeed in eating more healthily.

Eat breakfast

Breakfast is vital to renew yourself after your time asleep. If you skip breakfast, you will be more tempted to eat sugary cakes when you have your morning coffee or tea. A good breakfast is a bowl of unsweetened porridge and fruit or other non-sweetened cereal with a handful of nuts or egg, for protein.

Eat every two to three hours

To stop yourself overeating you need to keep your blood sugar at its normal level. You do this by having something small to eat 2 to 3 hours after you've eaten a meal. This keeps your blood sugar at a fairly even level and prevents craving and bingeing.

Eat something from each food group

Some so-called weight loss diets tell you to only eat a limited spectrum of food. For example: no carbs, only fat and protein. This may result in a rapid weight loss but at a price: your metabolism slows so that a very small amount of food can cause you to put back a large amount of weight. Make sure you have fruit and vegetables, lean protein and healthy fat at each meal.

Include lean protein at every meal

Protein helps you to feel full and satisfied. Have some at each meal and make sure you go for low fat meat, poultry with no skin and good fats such as avocado and olive oil.

Eat breakfast to lose weight

Could the secret of losing weight be having a healthy breakfast?

Too many people trying to lose weight choose not to have breakfast and believe that by so doing they will lose weight. This is not an effective way to lose weight. You must eat breakfast because after the hours since you ate the night before your blood sugar will have fallen and so until you raise it again your energy will be low and your ability to do things and think clearly will also be impaired too.

If you do something differently others things change too. Even changing what you have for breakfast will affect your health and well-being the rest of the day. Choose something nutritious such as porridge with fruit and yogurt with a handful of mixed seeds or nuts and you will be well set up for the day ahead with all your nutrients.

Having a good breakfast will have a beneficial effect on all parts of your life. You will be less likely to eat a sticky bun mid-morning and instead be satisfied with a healthy snack such as a piece of fruit and a few nuts.

Make the number one change in your life the resolution that from now on you will eat a healthy breakfast. Notice the difference in your life when you do this. Keep going until it becomes automatic: this may take up to twenty-one days before you reach for breakfast instead of rushing out fueled only by a cup of coffee.

Carbohydrates, do you need them?

———

Some diet schemes suggest eating low carbohydrates for rapid weight loss. Although you may find your weight drops rapidly when you do this, you may also find you begin to have massive craving for those very foods you've cut out of your diet.

For good health and well-being you need to eat a balanced diet which means eating from all the food groups: protein, fat and carbohydrates. The most important thing to remember is that within each of these groups there are good and not so good choices.

There are simple and complex carbohydrates. It's the simple ones you are better avoiding for good health and for weight loss too. These are foods with sugar or white flour in them. If you avoid any food with sugar such as jam, cakes, biscuits and sweetened breakfast cereals and instead eat foods which are naturally sweet such as fruit, or are made with whole grains such as whole-wheat bread or brown pasta, then you will be improving your health straight away and increasing your chances of becoming more healthy and attaining the weight you want.

Complex carbohydrates are found in fruits and vegetables. Every day cover at least half of your plate for lunch and dinner with vegetables. Eat them with herbs and spices instead of prepared sauces such as mayonnaise or ketchup.

Eat different vegetables every day. Some people suggest only eating starchy vegetables such as potatoes, rice, pasta in the middle of the day, not later. For your evening meal eat protein and vegetables only.

No pressure, just something you might like to try and find that not eating starchy carbohydrates in the evening means you may lose more weight.

Get the principles right and work out what's best for your body and your health.

Don't want to follow a strict eating programme?

If you want something to change then you have to do something differently.

While you eat too much unhealthy food and fail to exercise you will continue to be overweight and unhealthy. Your health and well-being will be affected. The outcome of not changing now will show sooner or later.

When you are eighty years old will you turn around and say, 'OK now I'm ready. Now I have the time to eat more healthily, do more exercise and find other ways to respond to emotions, instead of overeating.'

By then it could be too late to make a difference.

You already know the formula: 'Eat less, eat healthily and exercise more.'

What's stopping you?

What do you need to motivate yourself?

Will you have to restrict your food in unmanageable ways forever?

Some people find tremendous motivation from being accountable to a coach, a friend, a buddy or a support group, such as a slimming club.

Exercise for weight loss

A very important aspect of changing your weight is to move your body more by increasing the amount of exercise you take.

Instead of concentrating on losing fat it is beneficial to use your muscles more. By exercising more you are not only increasing your general fitness level you are also increasing your body's ability to burn fat. This is referred to as using calories. When you eat you take in calories and when you exercise you burn calories.

Unfortunately, many people don't take as much exercise as they could do because life has become more sedentary.

How can you increase the exercise you do?

You can:

- Take the stairs instead of elevator or lift
- Walk instead of using your car
- Cycle instead of walking
- Move more instead of sitting in front of a computer screen all day

Become more aware. Your weight is a balance between the calories you eat and the exercise you take. When your weight stays steady you have found the balance between these two. If you want to weigh less you must either burn more calories or eat less. It is preferable to do a bit of each by eating less and exercising more.

You must have muscles to burn more calories, the reason diets fail is when food calories are reduced but if exercise isn't increased, this ends up with a loss of muscle rather than loss of fat.

Unfortunately for those wanting to lose weight there is not only their sedentary lifestyle but also the foods high in sugar and therefore calories that are easy to eat but increase weight gain.

As well as increasing exercise and decreasing food calories it is advisable to adjust what you eat to foods that are lower in sugar and less processed, without additives. These will take longer to digest, leave you feeling satisfied for longer and so enable you to lose weight more easily.

Think natural when you decide what to eat and concentrate on foods which are as near as possible to their natural state. Eat as much organic as you can to be as healthy as possible and avoid ingestion of pesticides and other chemicals.

The best diet is one that you devise for yourself

What does that entail? It means learning about food and what is healthy. It means eating foods from each food group, protein, fat and carbohydrate: recognising when you have had enough and drinking plenty of water.

Most diets and slimming plans ask you to either eat meals as they prescribe or ask you to count calories or points. That's fine when you are well motivated and in control of where and what you eat.

But how do you manage when you go to a restaurant, to a friend's house or on holiday?

Do you really want someone telling you what to eat each day, or feeling guilty if you want another slice of bread?

Of course, the diets work, but only while you follow them. At some point you 'come off the diet' and your body rejoices by making you eat lots of the previously 'forbidden foods.' The result? You put back on all the weight you lost. I know from bitter experience this to be true!

- Get into the right mindset
- Trust yourself to make the right choices
- Learn about food and what your body needs
- Be adventurous and try different foods
- Always eat breakfast.
- Eat something every 2-3 hours to maintain your blood sugar level
- Have a variety of healthy foods available

- Forget about diets and calories
- Have snacks of complex carbohydrate and protein
- Fill up on fruit and vegetables

What's the very first thing to do? Think of how you would like to be when you are your ideal weight. Take a few minutes each day to sit quietly and imagine how you would like to look. The more you think about this image the more likely it will happen.

Weight loss – the importance of where you are.

Is it possible to lose weight wherever you are? Perhaps. But there may be better or worse places. Think about where and when you eat what you want to eat and yet lose weight compared with other places where you have a greater desire to eat the 'wrong' foods and your weight sours. In each of the situations listed below it is a common experience for some people to gain weight and for others to lose weight. What happens to you in each of the following situations and what could you do to bring the essence of when you lose weight to those situations when you commonly gain weight?

On holiday: You may be staying somewhere where all your meals are included such as a package tour which includes all you want to eat from a buffet. Or maybe you are catering for yourself or eating out in restaurants each day.

What happens? Do you fill your plate with unsuitable foods because it's all there and you want to get your money's worth?

Or do you remain conscious of the choices you have even in that situation and choose to have those foods which are suitable such as plenty of fruits and vegetables, low fat protein, wholemeal bread, and avoiding or limiting the number of cakes and puddings? Remember you always have a choice about what to put in your mouth and it is still possible to enjoy your holiday even if you are a bit more indulgent that you might be at home. Use the holiday time as a chance to eat healthily and come home feeling healthier than when you went.

At home: If you are the main food buyer then make sure you make healthy choices and avoid buying unhealthy foods 'just in case' you have visitors. If there are members of the family who want to eat high fat high sugar foods, let them

Visiting friends: It's fine to say 'no thank-you' when offered something which you don't want to eat or have had enough. If you like to have a second helping then start small and then you can have more. But watch for the usual culprits: have seconds of the food which is nearest to its natural state.

Going out for the day: Take some fruit or nuts with you to nibble on so you aren't tempted to eat too many unhealthy snacks.

Most of all remember that life is a balancing act. so long as you eat reasonably healthily 80% of the time don't be too stressed if you lapse for up to 20% of the time.

Eat less and exercise more

It's a simple matter of arithmetic. If you are not the size want to be then the balance between what you eat and how much you move is incorrect. Even if you believe that your diet is healthy then there will be another factor coming into play.

It may be because you eat healthy food, but you eat too much of it. You could reduce the size of your portions so that your intake is less or decide not to have a second helping. It is said you eat with your eyes, so you can fool yourself into believing you are eating more than you think by using a smaller plate and or piling high the low-calorie high bulk foods such as vegetables and salad.

Eat more fruit and vegetables and less high calorie foods. For example, eating avocado pear is a very healthy choice. it has good fat and plenty of vitamin E. But it has a lot of calories. You have to strike a balance weighting up how healthy a food is against how many calories it has.

To contrast you might know that a spoonful of sweet jam has fewer calories than half an avocado. Nutritionally it contains a large quantity of sugar so is not so beneficial for your health as an avocado even though it has less calories. Similarly with nuts which are good for your health, and contain healthy fat but are high in calories. So have some, perhaps a handful each day for your health but no more, to reduce your calorie intake.

Another way to lose weight is simply to write down everything you eat during the day. This enables you to discover ways to eat less but strangely enough even the act of recording what you eat seems to mean that you change your eating habits and as a result, lose your excess weight.

What is the best way to do this?

The easiest is walking. Walking every day. You may have your own preferences such as swimming, running, dancing, going to the gym, yoga and so on.

Do something that you love to do and can do regularly. You will notice the difference not only in your body but in your mind too.

If you are a person who spends a great deal of your time caring for others, whether this is in the course of your work or when you are at home with friends and family, you need to be a bit selfish too.

Particularly amongst people who are members of the caring professions such as doctors, nurses, health professionals, counsellers, coaches and mentors, there is a tendency to put other people's needs before your own. This may result in you feeling increased stress because you have the habit of dealing with other people's needs before your own. You probably believe that those people's needs are more important than yours.

It's OK to be selfish sometimes, especially when you are feeling very tired, exhausted, overwhelmed and wonder how you can continue to cope with your day-to-day activities. It's most important that you look after your own health and well-being needs and remember to look after yourself above all else. Although you may perceive this as being selfish and therefore not a good attribute to have, it is in fact something you must do to maintain your personal energy and well-being.

How can you do this? You can designate some time each week, or every day, however small that time turns out to be, that is just for you. You might, for example, take a few moments between tasks at work when you close your eyes and take a few slow deep breaths, in and out as you consciously let go of any areas of tension in your body. This exercise will take hardly any time and yet it will help to re-energise yourself for the rest of the day.

It's really important to also specify in advance a particular timeslot during which you can pursue something which you really enjoy. This might be something creative like writing, painting or taking photographs, or could be some physical exercise such as swimming, dancing or working out at the gym. Whatever it is it's really important to know that on that day there is some protected time just for you. It's too easy to dismiss your own needs and when asked to do a job for somebody else to always agree to it. But by designating specific time for your own needs, you can learn to be selfish at that time. When you are selfish in this way you will find you have increased energy and enthusiasm for all those things you do for other people.

Eat regularly

You may have tried to lose weight by skipping meals entirely. This doesn't work because your blood sugar drops and you begin to crave sugar and other simple carbohydrates. As a result, you will find yourself eating too much high calorie, high fat, unhealthy food and as a result your weight increases.

Eat healthily

If you think about what you're eating and try to make it as healthy as possible, without being fanatical, then you will have a much better chance of controlling your mindset and as a result, your weight.

This means a balanced diet, with plenty of fresh fruit and vegetables, low-fat protein, healthy fats such as olive oil and avocado, and plenty of complex carbohydrates. It also means cutting down on food containing sugar and white foods such as white flour, white rice and white pasta and eating instead more wholemeal foods

Relax frequently

If you tend to eat more when you are stressed take a few moments when you feel the tension building to close your eyes and take some slow breaths in as you breathe in relaxation and breathe out tension.

Listen to your body

Learn to listen to what your body tells you it needs at any time of the day and allow yourself to have whatever it seems to need even though at the same time being aware of the healthy guidelines mentioned above.

What is vital for your good health and well-being?

———

The answer is the food you eat. It has been said that you are what you eat, so if you eat junk food your body becomes full of junk and you become more prone to being overweight and the illnesses more common if you are obese.

Instead of junk if you eat healthful foods your body will become more fit and healthy. Here are the changes to make: to make sure you have plenty of vitamins and anti-oxidants to help your heart health and keep you looking younger.

Increase the amount of fruit and vegetables

Have at the recommended amount of at least five portions of fresh, frozen or tinned fruit of vegetables each day.

Try different colourful fruits and vegetables

Experiment with unusual fruits and vegetables and different ways to prepare them.

Have a salad or a piece of fruit with every meal

Reduce the saturated fat in your diet:

Eat more low-fat dairy foods such as cottage cheese and low-fat yoghurt to have enough calcium without increasing your saturated fat intake. Eat more healthy fats, such as olive oil and avocado and less saturated fat such as red meat and butter.

Eat less red meat and more while meat such as chicken and turkey.

Eat more good fats:

Olive oil is good to cook with and use on salads to make your diet more like a Mediterranean diet.

Avocados are full of vitamin E and good fats so make sure you have some regularly.

Increase your fish intake to have plenty of omega 3 fish oils from oily fish.

Think about your daily routine

Ask yourself if you are doing enough exercise. You know that in order to be fit and well you need to exercise your body, mind and spirit. Start with your body and discover ways to exercise it more.

Why is this so important?

Because people who don't take regular exercise are more likely to have a greater risk of becoming ill. If a large part of your working day is spent in front of a computer and you tend to grab something unhealthy to eat during the day, then think about your lifestyle and the need to introduce some more exercise into your daily life.

How could you do this?

You could: walk instead of driving or taking a train or bus. If this isn't practical then walk some of your journey.

Take a break during the day and get away from your desk to walk for ten minutes or more, either in a park, or along the streets nearby to get your circulation going and raise your heartbeat somewhat. Ideally thirty minutes of exercise such as walking would be hugely beneficial for your health and well-being.

What will you do differently to introduce some more movement into your life?

How can you make exercise a priority that you look forward to instead of a dreaded necessity that you try to avoid at all costs?

Think of something that can fit easily into your life without disrupting your normal routine.

Get a more positive approach to weight loss

Here are things you can do to manage your time and life more effectively and lose weight.

Plan your meals and snacks the previous evening

When you fail to plan it's easy to grab whatever you can when you feel hungry during the day. The most important meal is breakfast. You may have a habit of rushing out in the morning and grabbing a sweet bun with a milky coffee on the way to work. Instead to have some fruit with a bowl of muesli or porridge sprinkled with seeds or nuts, or an egg.

Avoid buying and eating 'ready meals'

If you eat badly because you don't have time to prepare suitable meals and instead buy ready meals with high fat and sugar content, then think again. Decide to prepare healthier options and freeze individual portions so you have several meals ready when you arrive home hungry.

Choose where you buy your ready meals

Sometimes buying ready-made food is the only option when you lead a busy life. However, choose where you buy these and look for healthy options especially choose meals with low fat and low sugar content, or make your own selection from a salad bar avoiding rich sauces and less healthy options.

Eating behaviour

Many people associate eating with various different emotions and for this reason they choose to eat more food to make them feel better, or happier, or comforted.

One of the easiest ways to change your eating behaviour is to eliminate any temptations. This is best done at the supermarket by not actually buying foods that are going to cause you a problem.

The secret of losing weight could be having a healthy breakfast.

Many people choose not to have breakfast and believe that by so doing they will lose weight. This is not ideal because after the hours since you ate the night before your blood sugar will have fallen and so until you raise it again your energy will be low and your ability to do things and think clearly will also be impaired.

When you do something differently others things change too. Even changing what you have for breakfast will affect your health and well-being the rest of the day.

Having a good breakfast has a beneficial effect on all parts of your life. You will be less likely to eat a sticky bun mid-morning and instead be satisfied with a healthy snack such as a piece of fruit and a few nuts.

Make the number one change in your life the resolution that from now on you will eat a healthy breakfast. Notice the difference in your life when you do this. Keep going until it becomes automatic: this may take up to twenty-one days before you reach for breakfast instead of rushing out, fuelled only by a cup of coffee.

Diets don't work

If you find after trying numerous "slimming diets", that diets don't work in the long term, then it's time to discover how to lose weight in a healthy and effective way. It's a combination of three things: what you eat, how much you exercise, and your mindset.

What do you eat?

You need to look at what food you eat, how much of it you have on your plate, and how often you eat it.

This means eating plenty of fruit and vegetables, lots of fish, low-fat meat and healthy oils from olives, nuts and avocados. You need to cut down on sugar and simple carbohydrates and increase complex carbohydrates such as brown rice, brown pasta and wholemeal bread.

Although on its own Mediterranean food may not result in significant weight loss, unless your current diet is full of sugar and fat, it will help you to become healthier.

The next thing is to notice how much you're eating. If you switch your diet to be healthier and don't lose weight then you need to reduce how much you put on your plate. Fill half your plate with salads and vegetables, a quarter with low-fat protein and a quarter with complex carbohydrates.

How much exercise?

Think about the amount of time you spend exercising and the sort of exercise you do.

For health and well-being you need to do some cardiovascular exercise for your heart health and some to stretch and exercise your joints. For example, you may want to take a brisk walk each day for about 30 minutes and do some yoga a couple of times a week. Not only will these exercises help your weight loss, but will also increase your sense of personal well being.

Your mindset

One of the most important things you need to engage with is your mindset, what you think about yourself now and the difference you expect when you achieve a healthy weight.

Success and confidence won't magically appear after you've lost weight. Do what you can do now to feel better about yourself and to increase your self-confidence.

Imagine yourself in the future, if you do nothing about your weight. As your 'future self' imagine looking back at the 'present you'.

What advice would the 'future you' give to the 'present you'? That is what to aim to put into practice!

Ways to lose weight without dieting

It is not as simple as saying that overweight people eat too much because there can be any number of psychological reasons that make people eat more than their body needs.

One of the most important skills to learn, when you want to lose weight, is being assertive. Saying no when you mean no. Not letting people persuade you to do things you don't want to do or eat what you don't want to eat. Recognise what it is that you want and avoid doing things just because you don't want to upset someone. Learning to say no is vitally important. Be selfish because that is the way to look after yourself and when you do, you will begin to eat more healthily and exercise more too.

Being overweight is more than just eating too much or exercising too little. It's hugely connected with mindset and using food as an emotional prop. So the most successful way to change your weight is to change your mind and find other ways apart from food to solve emotional challenges.

There is a discrepancy in the way society views obesity. Everywhere you look there are the latest diets, the best way to stick to your diet, the diet to get you slim for summer or for Christmas or for your holidays. All these diets are promoted as the only way to lose your excess weight and have your body transformed into a beautiful and probably rather unrealistic shape in just a few days.

On the other hand, if you keep on reading you will find articles and books that declare that diets don't work. Who or what can you believe?

If you weigh more than you would like, it is very tempting to attempt a quick fix. Half starve yourself for a few weeks and you will have the body of your dreams. No problem. Or is there? Here are the reasons why diets don't work:

- You may lose weight but it will be mainly fluid.
- When you restrict certain foods or drastically reduce the amount of food you eat you will, after a few days, crave those foods.
- It is bad for your general health to restrict what you eat to certain food groups and exclude others.
- When you cut down on the amount you eat your body goes into 'starvation mode' and tries to conserve both energy and food stores as fat.
- It will manage on less food so that when you reach your desired weight and increase what you eat your weight will increase rapidly again and is likely to be higher than the original weight.
- Life happens even when you are trying to lose weight: it is extremely difficult to have a social life and stick rigidly to any eating programme for a sustained length of time.

You have to:

- Learn again what hunger feels like and how to satisfy it.
- Not satisfy your hunger with calorie dense foods such as those containing excessive sugar and fat and refined carbohydrates.
- Enjoy eating more healthy food.
- Discover new flavours.
- Eat a balance of protein, carbohydrates and fat.
- Look at ways to cut down or remove from your food anything with sugar and high saturated fat content.
- Stop turning to food when you are upset or depressed, instead find other ways to deal with these emotions.

Weight loss and good intentions

However good your intentions for keeping to a healthy diet and progressing in your weight loss journey to become the weight you truly want to be, there are days when things just don't work out well.

Even though you plan to cut down on the amount of white flour and then see and smell the aroma of freshly baked bread with sunflower seeds, (so it must be healthy!) and honey (could be better than white sugar?!) You meant to eat just a slice but the taste was so delicious that before you know it most of the loaf has disappeared and your stomach feels rather bloated and full.

We've all been tempted haven't we and sometimes given in to the cravings. So the secret is not to give up but to pick yourself up, dust yourself down and start again: eating healthily, plenty of fresh wholesome fruits and vegetables, whole grains, lean proteins, some healthy fat from avocado, olives, nuts and oily fish, and some low fat dairy foods such as yoghurt and cottage cheese. You will soon be back on track once more!

As always keep your goals in your mind and don't give up if occasionally you slip off the path you are on. If you are following the advice given here rather than a very strict diet regime then you will lose weight because you are treating your body well and you are keeping your mindset positive too. Being in the right mindset is the number one important thing to aim for. Get into it by practicing regular relaxation and visualising how you will be when you reach your desired weight.

How to regain the weight you lost

If you are fed up with diet routines and think that the easiest thing to do would be to stop all this bother with weight loss and just eat whatever takes your fancy, especially if it's sweet and fatty.

You've had enough of dietary instructions and paying out so much each week to the club leader.

You throw away the diet books and the slimming club rules and regulations and have a massive binge and want to continue in this way and forget about ever getting slimmer.

You've made up your mind that diets are the only way and when you have a special occasion, you'll go on a crash diet and lose what has to be lost.

Here are some ways to regain any weight lost extremely quickly:

Skip meals and then overeat

Remain convinced that the only witness to lose weight is to stop eating, so never eat anything until the evening, then it won't matter how much food you eat or what sort of food it is.

Keep away from healthy food

Don't bother with anything that sounds healthy, it can't possibly do you any good, just keep eating as much sugary, fatty and fast food as you possibly can.

Most of all don't make any attempt at having a balanced diet, but never eat fresh fruit or vegetables. Have a fry up breakfast every day and put plenty of salt all over your food and keep away from anything wholemeal.

Don't relax, ever. Don't find out what relaxation means. If you feel tension in your back on your shoulders or suffer from frequent headaches make sure that you take plenty of painkillers and see your GP regularly for prescription for more of the same.

Only do what others do. If your friends all like eating junk food then follow along at and do the same. A burger and chips will fill a gap for you and you can be sure that within an hour two if not sooner you will be craving for more of the same and quite soon your weight will begin to increase too.

Of course, all of the above will have the rapid effect of increasing your weight. If that's not what you truly what you want then just reverse what is suggested and the opposite will happen. Your excess weight will gradually come off, your general health will improve and you will slowly move towards a healthy weight.

How to get your weight loss back on track

Most people, whatever they are trying to do, have days when things work very well and other days when they feel stuck. When this happens remember it is a temporary phase. It will pass and you will achieve a healthy weight.

Sometimes even the most motivated person finds that things start to go wrong. If you have spent several weeks eating healthy food, doing regular exercise and becoming much healthier and then have a day or two when you seem to forget all your good intentions. During that time, you eat too much unhealthy food. As a result, your weight goes up, you feel fat and bloated and begin to think that you will never achieve the healthy weight you're aiming for.

Please don't give up. It's a common experience in the journey of change to feel as if you have gone off track or as though you will never achieve what you were trying to accomplish.

The most important thing is to recognise this and do what is necessary to quickly get back on track.

Plan what you will do tomorrow

Even though you feel as though all is lost, tomorrow is another day and you can plan carefully what to eat and drink. Maybe you need to overhaul your food supplies or decide to go out for lunch at a local healthy restaurant.

Get rid of unhealthy foods

If packets of unhealthy food have invaded your fridge and food cupboard, get rid of them and replace what you throw away with plenty of fresh fruit and vegetables, low fat protein and wholemeal carbohydrates.

By not having unhealthy food at home you won't be tempted. This will encourage you to eat healthy food and in doing so change your behaviour patterns.

Drink plenty of water:

Since people are mostly made of water, you need to make sure you drink plenty of plain water to keep your body hydrated. Notice what you drink and replace soft drinks full of additives with water or low-calorie squash, herb teas and decaffeinated coffee.

Take a different sort of exercise

If you've forgotten to exercise recently then start again:

- Go out of your front door and walk down the street for 10 or 15 minutes.
- Join a new exercise class or start to do some yoga.
- Put on some lively music and dance around your home until you feel yourself becoming hot and sweaty.

Get some support from a sympathetic friend

Find a friend who is also trying to change their lifestyle and give each other the support that you both need.

Become energetic and motivated once again

You will find that when you get back on track after a lapse that more motivation will very quickly achieve the result you want to accomplish. What is important to realise is that most people, whatever they are trying to achieve, have days when things work very well and other days when they feel stuck. When this happens remember it is a temporary phase and it will pass and you will be back on track to achieving a healthy weight, before you know it.

How to maintain your weight loss

You have ever had the experience of being so-called successful at losing weight following being a member of a slimming club for a few months, only to re-gain all the weight that she lost when you stop attending regularly.

It seems as if it is almost like a plot to keep you paying to keep on going to the slimming club otherwise you find that you can't maintain your weight loss.

So, in order to maintain the success you feel you've add you need to do more than just go regularly to a slimming club or follow a diet in a newspaper.

It's about changing your mindset about your weight and realising that diets on their own won't work. Yes, if you follow what is written, or what you're told and you will lose some weight. However, the weight is in many and most cases regained very quickly once you decide you're going back to a "normal" diet.

If diets don't work, then what can you do to be the way that you would like to be, and be healthy too.

Eat regularly.

You may have tried to lose weight by skipping meals entirely. This doesn't work because your blood sugar level drops and you begin to crave lots of sugar and other simple carbohydrates. As a result he will probably find yourself eating too much high calorie, high fat, unhealthy food and as a result find it anyway kudos goes back on very quickly.

Eat healthily.

If you think about is actually what you're eating and try to make your diet is healthy as possible, without being fanatical, then you will have a much better chance at being able to control your weight by controlling your mindset.

Eating healthily means having a balanced diet, eating plenty of fresh fruit and vegetables, low-fat protein, healthy fats such as olive oil and avocado, and plenty of complex carbohydrates. It also means cutting right down on food containing sugar and white foods such as white flour, white rice and white pasta and eating instead more wholemeal foods

Relax frequently.

If you tend to eat more when you feel stressed take a few moments when you feel the stress building to close your eyes and take some slow breaths in as you breathe in relaxation and breathe out any tension.

Listen to your body.

Learn to listen to what your body tells you it needs at any time of the day and allow yourself to have whatever it seems to need even though at the same time being aware of the healthy guidelines mentioned above.

Exercise

If you want to lose weight than it's most important to exercise regularly.

What is regular exercising? It means three things:

- Moving your body so that your heart rate increases.
- Maintaining that for at least 30 minutes every day.
- Using more calories exercising than you take in with your food.
- Stretching your muscles and joints to keep mobility.

Why is it important to exercise so that your heart rate increases? It's because your heart is the most important muscle in your body and it needs to be strong so that if necessary you can respond to danger by moving quickly, or running away from it. If you never exercise your heart muscle may become weak.

The most effective and easiest way to achieve this is to walk briskly every day for 30 minutes. Some people prefer jogging or playing golf and either of these would be fine.

However, the most important thing is that your heartbeat is raised for at least 30 minutes. This is aerobic exercise. Other sorts of exercise are useful too and are known as anaerobic exercise. With these you have periods of activity and periods of rest. Examples are: playing tennis, football or basketball.

Eating provides calories or energy that you need to keep your body functioning well. Unfortunately, you may be taking in more calories in your food than you need for this and so you put on weight.

Exercise increases how many calories you use each day. So doing more exercise than you do now will result in weight loss. If you do intensive exercise such as marathon running you may be surprised at how many calories you can eat and still lose weight.

Unfortunately, too much weight loss advice is based on eating less or counting what goes into your body rather than being about the balance between what goes in and what is used.

Part of the ageing process is that your joints and muscles become stiffer because you do less exercise. Any exercise is good but particularly beneficial are exercises that involve stretching your muscles and moving your joints on a regular basis. The perfect way to do this is to practice yoga regularly.

Walking is the easiest way to exercise

You can do it every day wherever you are and fit it around work and social commitments without the need for any special equipment, with or without other people.

Walk when you can, instead of driving.

Take the stairs whenever possible. If you walk outside in fresh air, so much better.

As well as walking consider yoga and swimming as other ways for positive health and well-being.

Exercise is vital so do some regularly.

It will keep you well for longer, enable your heart to beat more strongly, your joints will be more mobile and your body flexible and better able to cope with whatever happens. If you are unlucky to become ill you will be fit enough to heal more quickly and effectively.

More about exercise

The weather is bad, it's raining or snowing or extremely windy. Perhaps at another time of the year it's too hot and too humid. Maybe you are tired or have eaten too much or drunk too much. Whatever you use as your excuse you decide you haven't got the energy or motivation to exercise today, or tomorrow or next week or next month. So your exercise routine fails again and you decide you can get along very nicely, thank you very much, without doing any exercise.

Yet there is a reason to keep going, there is a reason to re-motivate yourself to exercise on a regular basis, whatever the weather, however tired you feel. It's a matter of looking after yourself.

Why do you need to look after yourself?

To have a full, long and healthy life.

Why should you include exercise?

Because part of being healthy is to have limbs and joints that move, to have a body that is as flexible as possible for your own body shape, age and ability and to keep blood circulating into all the nooks and crannies of your body. When you keep fit through exercise you will maintain a healthier body weight too than if you sit around and never exercise.

What can you do instead of excuses?

Dress appropriately, if your exercise involves going outside. There is no such thing as bad weather only the wrong clothes. You can exercise indoors or outside as you wish. You can vary the type of exercise and how strenuously you do the exercise.

If you are unwell or feelings extra tired do something gentler than when you are bounding with energy.

However, the most important thing is to do something. Walking, swimming, yoga, dancing and T'ai Chi are all forms of exercise that you can do gently or more vigorously. Pick several different forms of exercise but a minimum would be to walk for thirty minutes at least five days a week. This can be divided into three shorter bursts of ten minutes if necessary.

Commit to do something on a regular basis.

Do whatever you must do to keep motivated. You could get a friend to exercise with you but whatever you do you must fit exercise into your daily routine without fail.

Unhealthy versus healthy

What is unhealthy eating?

Some foods have very little nutritional value and are best avoided especially if they form the bulk of what you eat. These are foods with a lot of additives and processed foods. They include foods containing white sugar and white flour. If you tend to eat a lot of junk food full of additives, you are not giving your body the fuel it needs to function efficiently.

What is healthy eating?

You need to eat healthy food because as the saying goes: 'you are what you eat.'

Foods in their natural unprocessed state tend to be healthier and more beneficial for your body. These include fruits, vegetables and lean meats. All fish, especially oily fish, such as salmon, trout, mackerel and herring, supply your body with omega 3 oils, are good for the heart and should be eaten several times each week.

Healthy food includes beans, pulses, seeds and nuts. These provide healthy fats but also protein and vitamins necessary for body repair.

Why eat more healthily?

If you want to live as long and as healthily as you can then what you eat is an important factor. If you are unfortunate enough to be ill then you will have a strong immune system and be better able to resist infection or fight it if you need to.

Eating healthily is part of your vital need to care for yourself: body, mind and spirit. Your body needs the nutrition that you provide from good quality nutrients instead of highly processed food.

You are more likely to maintain a healthy body weight when you eat healthily. You are less likely to gain the excessive weight that follows eating food with low nutritional value.

Start today, think more about what you are eating and about the body you are trying to keep in as good a shape and state of health as you can. Not only yours but your family's too, if you are the one who shops and cooks for them. Keep them in tiptop health.

Finally

If you are fed up with your life, your weight or your body, then it's time to do something to make a difference.

Don't miss out!

Visit the website below and you can sign up to receive emails whenever Susan Kersley publishes a new book. There's no charge and no obligation.

https://books2read.com/r/B-A-EFNC-FBFT

BOOKS 2 READ

Connecting independent readers to independent writers.

Did you love *Weight Loss Success*? Then you should read *Mind Over Weight*[1] by Susan Kersley!

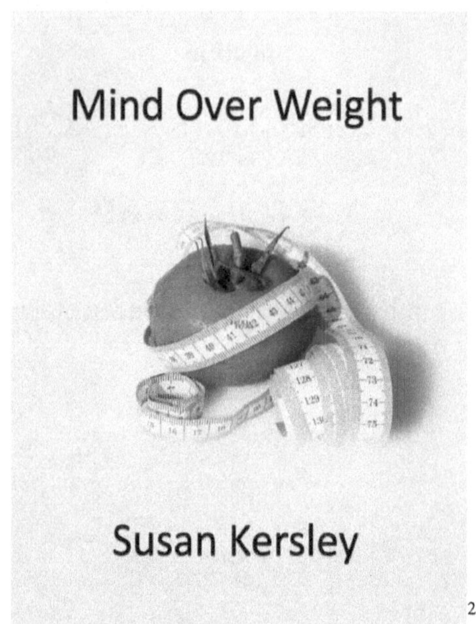

[2]

In order to reach a healthy weight, it's important to change your mindset. Beliefs about food may need to change. In the long term, diets don't work. Eating more healthily and increasing exercise is vital, but your mindset is too.

Read more at https://susankersley.co.uk.

---

1. https://books2read.com/u/mleWKZ

2. https://books2read.com/u/mleWKZ

Also by Susan Kersley

Books about Weight Management
Change Your Mind, Change Your Weight
Mind Over Weight
Weight Loss Success

Books for Doctors
Critical Mistakes Nearly Every Doctor Makes
Simple Ways to Meet the Challenges of Working as a Doctor

Retirement Books
Get Ready for Retirement
Retire and Let Go of Myths
Retire and Look After Yourself
Retire and Communicate
Retire and Decide What to Do
Life After Work
Retire to a Life Transition

Self-help Books
How to Have a Balanced Life
15 Ways to Change Your Life

Standalone
Lifestyle Coaching for Doctors
ABC of Change for Doctors
Life After Medicine
Prescription for Time
Pills and Pillboxes
Prescription for Change
69 Easy Ways to Change Your life
Mary and the Photograph
More Time for You Now!
Enjoy your retirement
Coping with New year Resolutions
More than 80 ways for a Busy Doctor to Have More Time
Connection Deception

Watch for more at https://susankersley.co.uk.

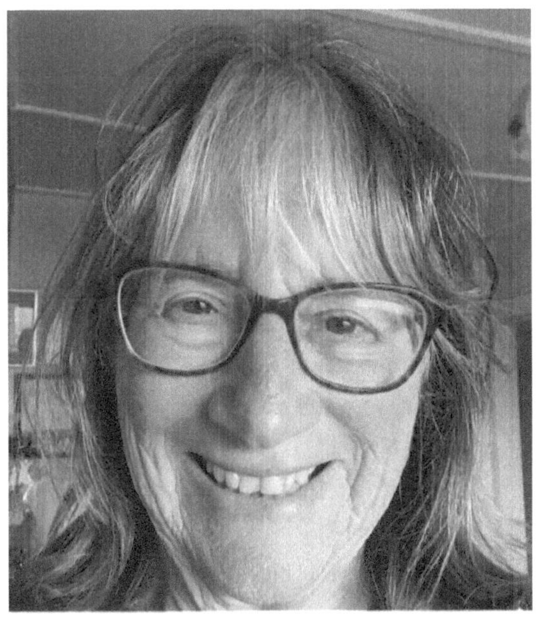

About the Author

If you enjoyed this book, **please take a moment to leave a review.** I would really appreciate a review on the website from which you downloaded or bought this book.

Reviews are so important for independent authors.

Thank you very much.

I live by the sea in Cornwall, UK. I've written personal development and self-help books for doctors and others, books about retirement and novels.

I was a doctor for thirty years and did something else.

After attending a workshop based on Louise Hay's book 'You Can Heal Your Life', I trained to be a Louise Hay workshop leader. I did this in 1999 in San Diego and for several years ran workshops in Cornwall, UK. The aim of these workshops was to enable participants to understand themselves better and then find how to move forward more positively in life.

I read an article about Coaching, so I trained with CoachU. In 2000 I had an epiphany and realised that as a doctor, gave me useful and special insights and life experience about what life is like as a doctor, so I focussed on coaching doctors.

I wrote an article called 'Is there life after medicine?' for the BMJ hoping that it would be published in 'Personal View.' However even though the panel rejected it I was contacted by and later met Rhona MacDonald, the editor of Career Focus, part of the British Medical Journal. She was very interested in what I was doing and encouraged me to write a series of articles about Life Coaching and how it can enable doctors to have a life. As a result, I wrote each month about how doctors could have more time and better work-life balance. These articles were published in the British Medical Journal over the years 2000-2005 and eventually evolved into books for doctors: 'Prescription for Change - for Doctors who want a life' and 'ABC of Change for Doctors.' 'Life after Medicine - for Doctors who want a trouble-free transition' was published later.

Since then I've also written and published various books, eBooks and audiobooks: personal development books for doctors, self-help books, and novels.

Now retired from Coaching, I'm updating my books and writing more.

Read more at https://susankersley.co.uk.

www.ingramcontent.com/pod-product-compliance
Lightning Source LLC
Chambersburg PA
CBHW031131160726
47989CB00017B/2886